Medicinal Herbs

To Boosts Immune
System Plus Prevent
Disease

Bilingual Edition
English Germany

by

Jannah Firdaus Mediapro

2021

Prologue

Medicinal Herbs to Boosts Immune System Plus Prevent Disease Bilingual Edition In English and Germany Languange.

Feeding your body with certain foods like fruit and vegetables may help keep your immune system strong. If you're looking for ways to prevent winter colds, virus attack and the flu.

Your first step should be a visit to your local grocery store. Plan your meals to include these powerful immune system boosters.

Wenn Sie Ihren Körper mit bestimmten Lebensmitteln wie Obst und Gemüse füttern, kann dies dazu beitragen, Ihr Immunsystem zu stärken. Wenn Sie nach Möglichkeiten suchen, um Erkältungen im Winter, Virenbefall und Grippe vorzubeugen.

Ihr erster Schritt sollte ein Besuch in Ihrem örtlichen Lebensmittelgeschäft sein. Planen Sie Ihre Mahlzeiten mit diesen leistungsstarken Boostern des Immunsystems.

Medicinal Herbs to Boosts Immune System English Version

Feeding your body certain foods like fruit and vegetables may help keep your immune system strong. If you're looking for ways to prevent winter colds, virus attack and the flu.

Your first step should be a visit to your local grocery store. Plan your meals to include these powerful immune system boosters.

1. Citrus Fruits

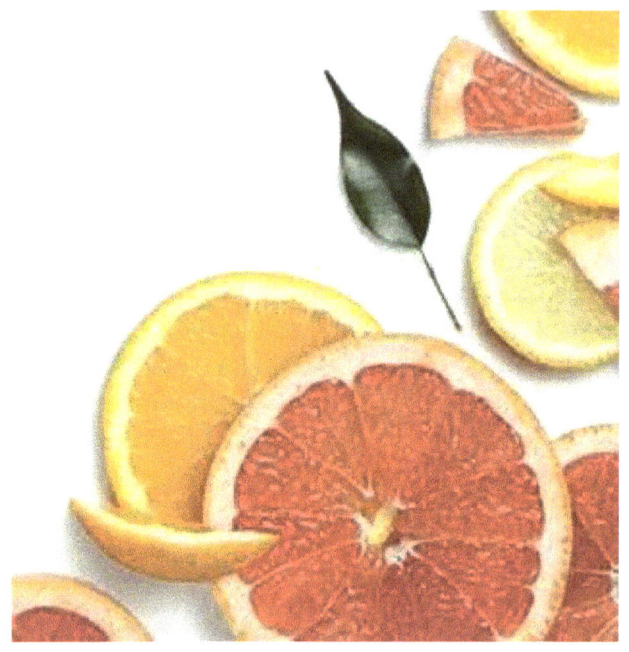

Most people turn to vitamin C after they've caught a cold. That's because it helps build up your immune system. Vitamin C is thought to increase the production of white blood cells. These are

Because your body doesn't produce or store it, you need daily vitamin C for continued health. Almost all citrus fruits are high in vitamin C. With such a variety to choose from, it's easy to add a squeeze of this vitamin to any meal.

2. Red Bell Peppers

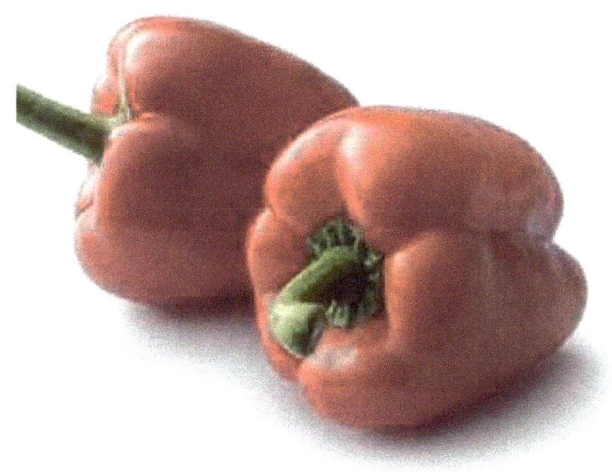

If you think citrus fruits have the most vitamin C of any fruit or vegetable, think again. Ounce for ounce, red bell peppers contain twice as much vitamin C as citrus. They're also a rich source of beta carotene. Besides boosting your immune system, vitamin C may help maintain healthy skin. Beta carotene helps keep your eyes and skin healthy.

3. Broccoli

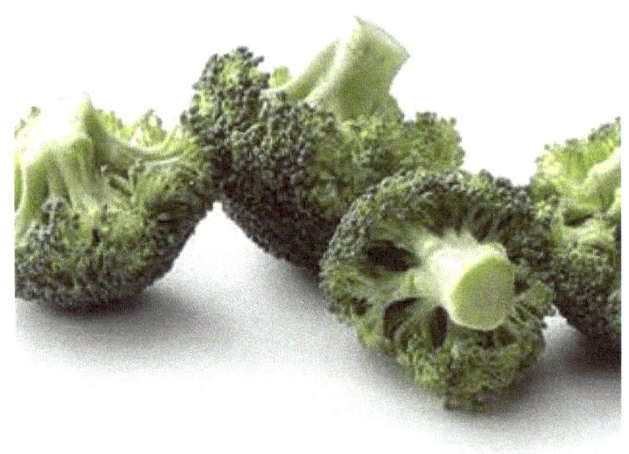

Broccoli is supercharged with vitamins and minerals. Packed with vitamins A, C, and E, as well as many other antioxidants and fiber.

Broccoli is one of the healthiest vegetables you can put on your table. The key to keeping its power intact is to cook it as little as possible — or better yet, not at all.

4. Garlic

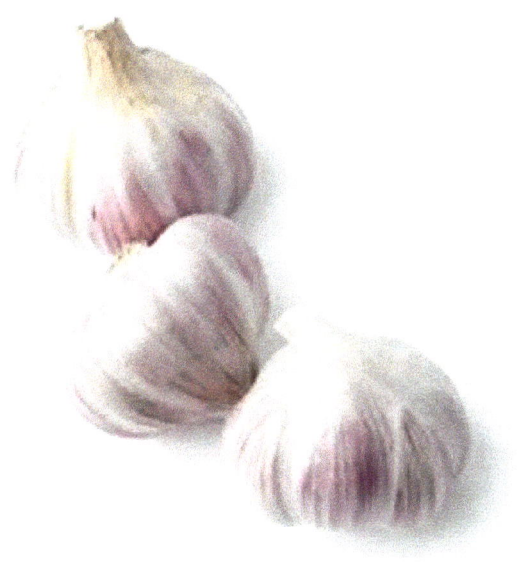

Garlic is found in almost every cuisine in the world. It adds a little zing to food and it's a must-have for your health. Early civilizations recognized its value in fighting infections.

According to the National Center for Complementary and Integrative, garlic may also help lower blood pressure and slow down hardening of the arteries. Garlic's immune-boosting properties seem to come from a heavy concentration of sulfur-containing compounds, such as allicin.

5. Ginger

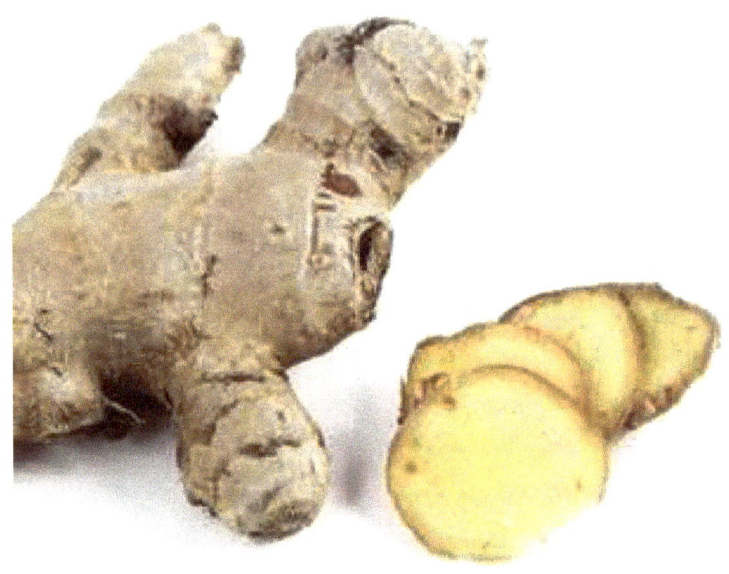

Ginger is another ingredient many turn to after getting sick. Ginger may help decrease inflammation, which can help reduce a sore throat and other inflammatory illnesses. Ginger may also help decrease nausea.

While it's used in many sweet desserts, ginger packs some heat in the form of gingerol, a relative of capsaicin.

Ginger may help decrease chronic pain and may possess cholesterol-lowering properties, according to recent animal research.

6. Spinach

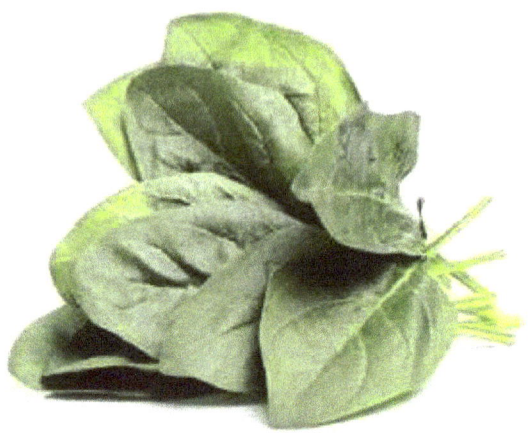

Spinach made our list not just because it's rich in vitamin C. It's also packed with numerous antioxidants and beta carotene, which may increase the infection-fighting ability of our immune systems.

Similar to broccoli, spinach is healthiest when it's cooked as little as possible so that it retains its nutrients. However, light cooking enhances its vitamin A and allows other nutrients to be released from oxalic acid.

7. Yogurt

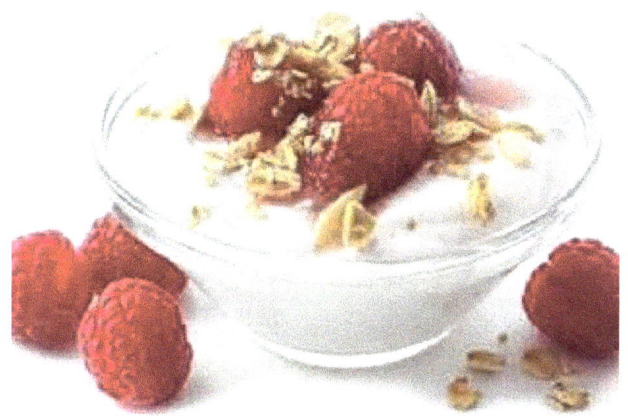

Look for yogurts that have "live and active cultures" printed on the label, like Greek yogurt.

These cultures may stimulate your immune system to help fight diseases.

Try to get plain yogurts rather than the kinds that are preflavored and loaded with sugar.

You can sweeten plain yogurt yourself with healthy fruits and a drizzle of honey instead.

Yogurt can also be a great source of vitamin D, so try to select brands fortified with vitamin D.

Vitamin D helps regulate the immune system and is thought to boost our body's natural defenses against diseases.

8. Almonds

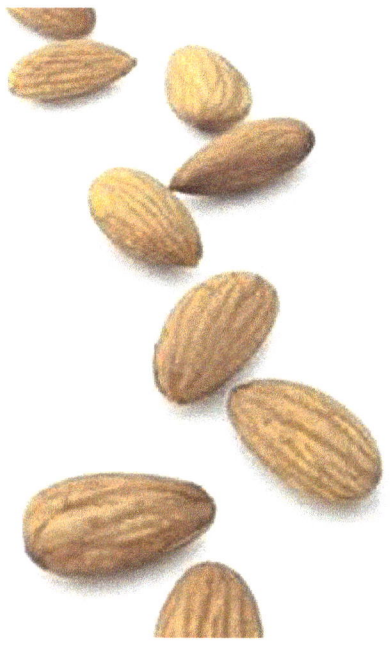

When it comes to preventing and fighting off colds, vitamin E tends to take a backseat to vitamin C.

However, vitamin E is key to a healthy immune system. It's a fat-soluble vitamin, meaning it requires the presence of fat to be absorbed properly.

Nuts, such as almonds, are packed with the vitamin and also have healthy fats.

A half-cup serving, which is about 46 whole, shelled almonds, provides nearly 100 percent of the recommended daily amount of vitamin E.

9. Turmeric

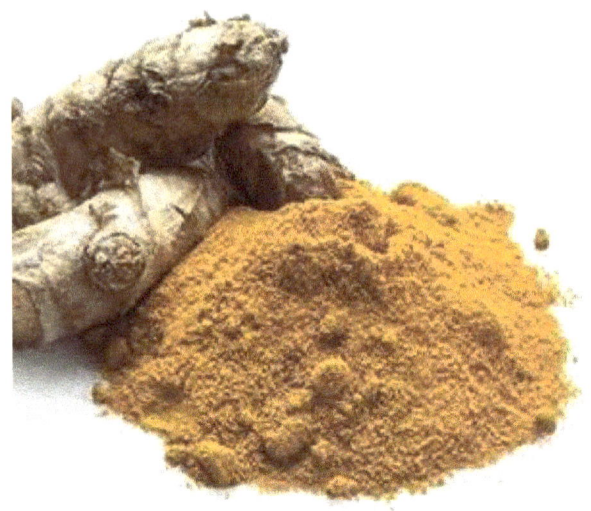

You may know turmeric as a key ingredient in many curries. But this bright yellow, bitter spice has also been used for years as an anti-inflammatory in treating both osteoarthritis and rheumatoid arthritis.

Also, research shows that high concentrations of curcumin, which gives turmeric its distinctive color, can help decrease exercise-induced muscle damage.

10. Green Tea

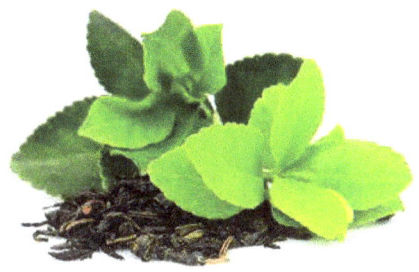

Both green and black teas are packed with flavonoids, a type of antioxidant. Where green tea really excels is in its levels of epigallocatechin gallate, or EGCG, another powerful antioxidant. EGCG has been shown to enhance immune function.

The fermentation process black tea goes through destroys a lot of the EGCG. Green tea, on the other hand, is steamed and not fermented, so the EGCG is preserved. Green tea is also a good source of the amino acid L-theanine. L-theanine may aid in the production of germ-fighting compounds in your T-cells.

11. Papaya

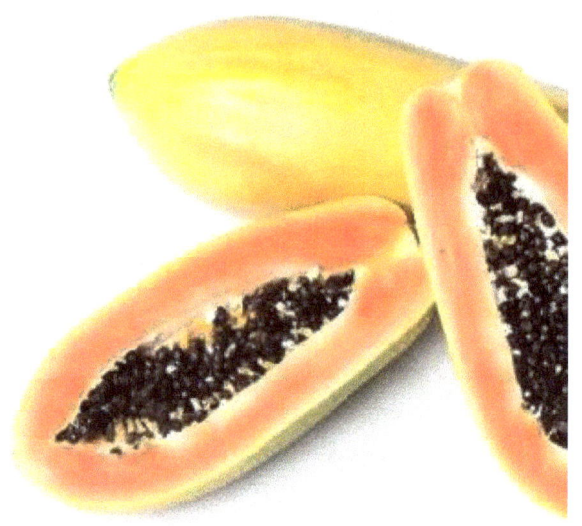

Papaya is another fruit loaded with vitamin C. You can find 224 percent of the daily recommended amount of vitamin C in a single papaya.

Papayas also have a digestive enzyme called papain that has anti-inflammatory effects.

Papayas have decent amounts of potassium, B vitamins, and folate, all of which are beneficial to your overall health.

12. Kiwi

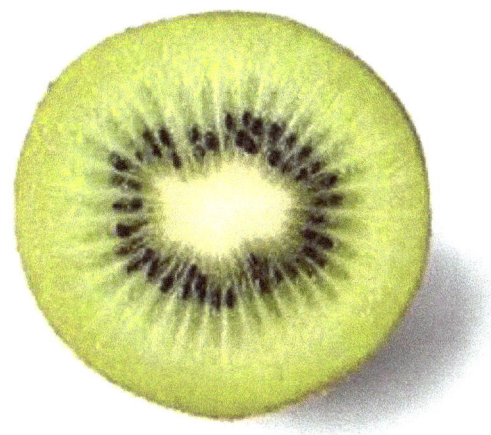

Like papayas, kiwis are naturally full of a ton of essential nutrients, including folate, potassium, vitamin K, and vitamin C.

Vitamin C boosts white blood cells to fight infection, while kiwi's other nutrients keep the rest of your body functioning properly.

13. Sunflower seeds

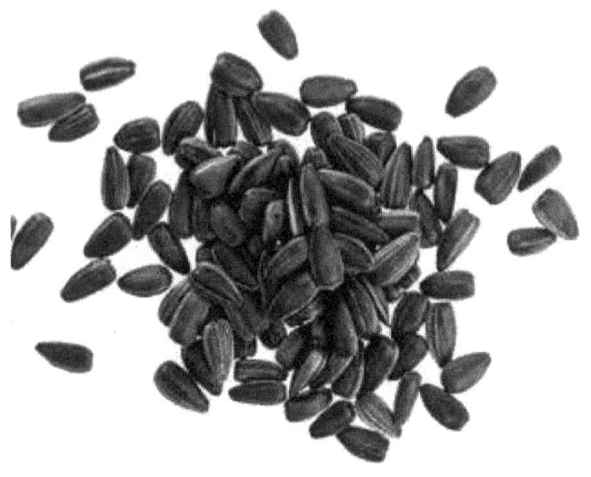

Sunflower seeds are full of nutrients, including phosphorous, magnesium, and vitamin B-6. They're also incredibly high in vitamin E, a powerful antioxidant.

Vitamin E is important in regulating and maintaining immune system function. Other foods with high amounts of vitamin E include avocados and dark leafy greens.

14. Oregano

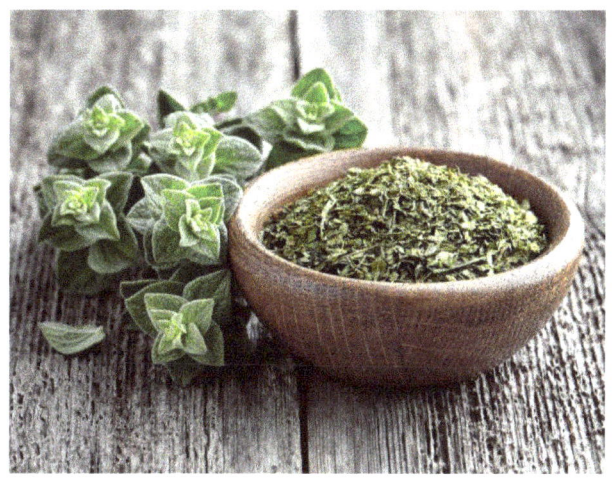

Oregano is a popular herb in the mint family that's known for its impressive medicinal qualities. Its plant compounds, which include carvacrol, offer antiviral properties.

In a test-tube study, both oregano oil and isolated carvacrol reduced the activity of murine norovirus (MNV) within 15 minutes of exposure.

NV is highly contagious and the primary cause of stomach flu in humans. It is very similar to human norovirus and used in scientific studies because human norovirus is notoriously difficult to grow in laboratory settings

Oregano oil and carvacrol have also been shown to exhibit antiviral activity against herpes simplex virus type-1 (HSV-1).

Rotavirus, a common cause of diarrhea in infants and children; and respiratory syncytial virus (RSV), which causes respiratory infections.

15. Echinacea

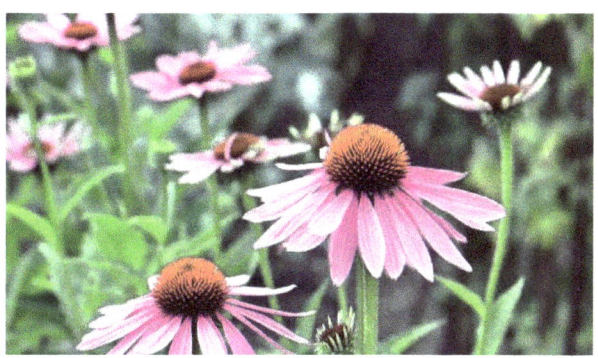

Echinacea is one of the most popularly used ingredients in herbal medicine due to its impressive health-promoting properties. Many parts of the plant, including its flowers, leaves, and roots, are used for natural remedies.

In fact, *Echinacea purpurea*, a variety that produces cone-shaped flowers, was used by Native Americans to treat a wide array of conditions, including viral infections.

Several test-tube studies suggest that certain varieties of echinacea, including *E. pallida*, *E. angustifolia*, and *E. purpurea*, are particularly effective at fighting viral infections like herpes and influenza.

Notably, *E. purpurea* is thought to have immune-boosting effects as well, making it particularly useful for treating viral infections.

16. Ginseng

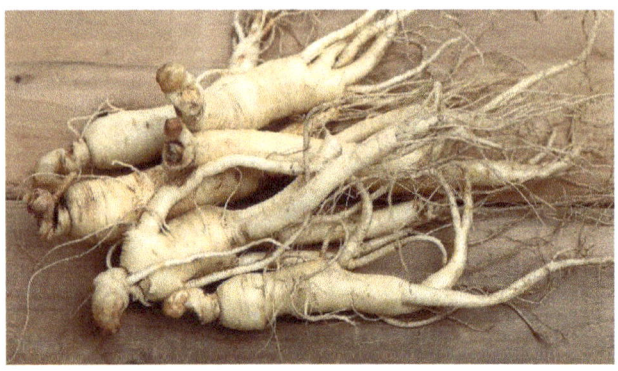

Ginseng, which can be found in Korean and American varieties, is the root of plants in the *Panax* family.

Long used in traditional Chinese medicine, it has been shown to be particularly effective at fighting viruses.

In animal and test-tube studies, Korean red ginseng extract has exhibited significant effects against RSV, herpes viruses, and hepatitis A.

Plus, compounds in ginseng called ginsenosides have antiviral effects against hepatitis B, norovirus, and coxsackieviruses,

Which are associated with several serious diseases — including an infection of the brain called meningoencephalitis.

17. Peppermint

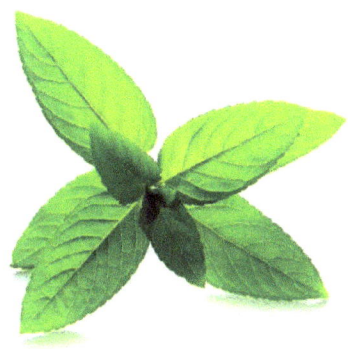

Peppermint is known to have powerful antiviral qualities and commonly added to teas, extracts, and tinctures meant to naturally treat viral infections.

Its leaves and essential oils contain active components, including menthol and rosmarinic acid, which have antiviral and anti-inflammatory activity.

In a test-tube study, peppermint-leaf extract exhibited potent antiviral activity against respiratory syncytial virus (RSV) and significantly decreased levels of inflammatory compounds.

18. Sambucus

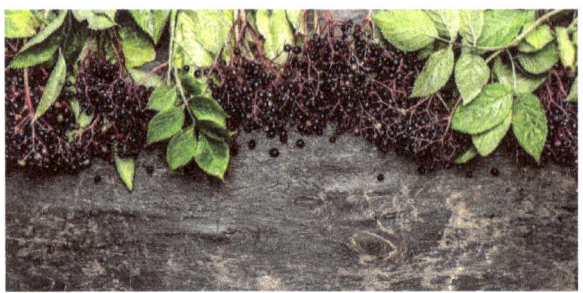

Sambucus is a family of plants also called elder. Elderberries are made into a variety of products, such as elixirs and pills that are used to naturally treat viral infections like the flu and common cold.

A study in mice determined that concentrated elderberry juice suppressed influenza virus replication and stimulated immune system response.

What's more, in a review of 4 studies in 180 people, elderberry supplements were found to substantially reduce upper respiratory symptoms caused by viral infections.

19. Licorice

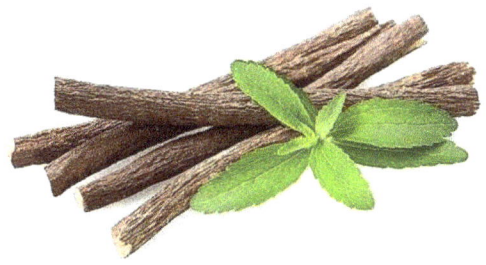

Licorice has been used in traditional Chinese medicine and other natural practices for centuries. Glycyrrhizin, liquiritigenin, and glabridin are just some of the active substances in licorice that have powerful antiviral properties.

Test-tube studies demonstrate that licorice root extract is effective against HIV, RSV, herpes viruses, and severe acute respiratory syndrome-related coronavirus (SARS-CoV), which causes a serious type of pneumonia.

20. Astragalus

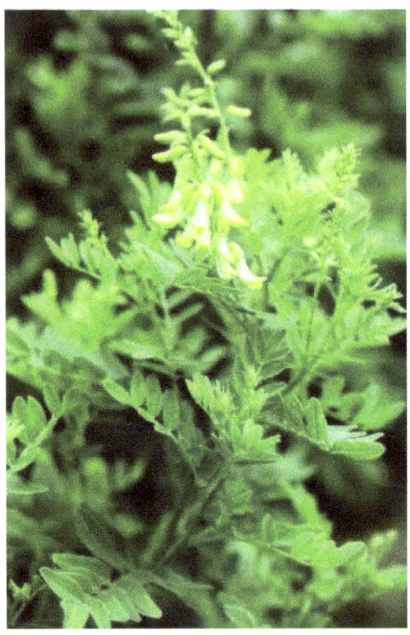

Astragalus is a flowering herb popular in traditional Chinese medicine. It boasts Astragalus polysaccharide (APS), which has significant immune-enhancing and antiviral qualities.

Test-tube and animal studies show that astragalus combats herpes viruses, hepatitis C, and avian influenza H9 virus.

Plus, test-tube studies suggest that APS may protect human astrocyte cells, the most abundant type of cell in the central nervous system, from infection with herpes.

21. Dandelion

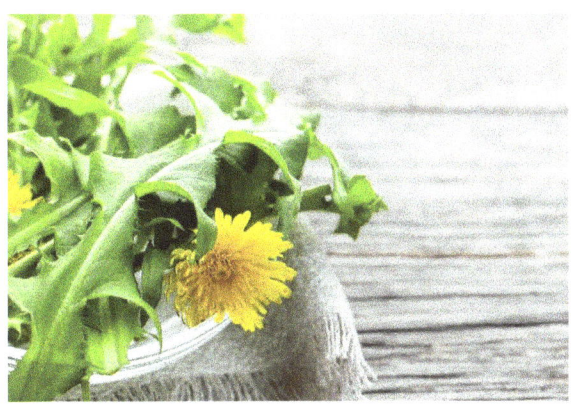

Dandelions are widely regarded as weeds but have been studied for multiple medicinal properties, including potential antiviral effects. Test-tube research indicates that dandelion may combat hepatitis B, HIV, and influenza.

Moreover, one test-tube study noted that dandelion extract inhibited the replication of dengue, a mosquito-borne virus that causes dengue fever.

This disease, which can be fatal, triggers symptoms like high fever, vomiting, and muscle pain,

22. Sage

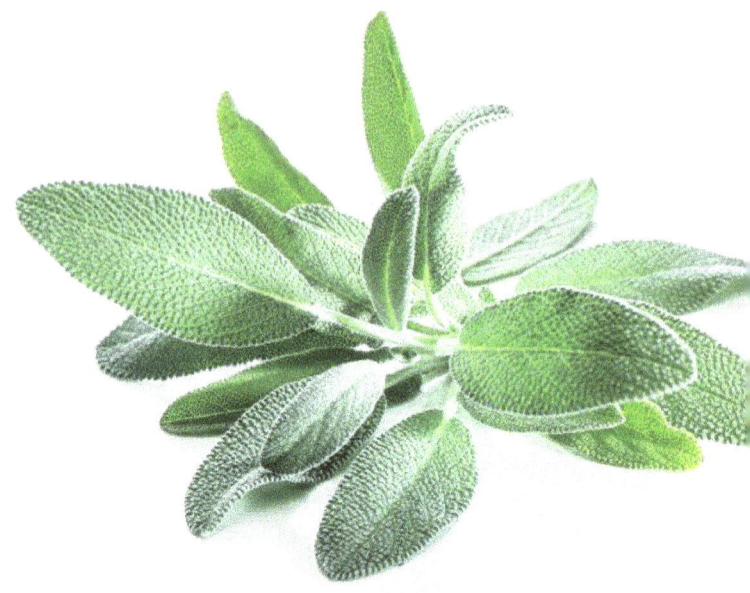

Also a member of the mint family, sage is an aromatic herb that has long been used in traditional medicine to treat viral infections.

The antiviral properties of sage are mostly attributed to compounds called safficinolide and sage one, which are found in the leaves and stem of the plant.

Test-tube research indicates that this herb may fight human immunodeficiency virus type 1 (HIV-1), which can lead to AIDS. In one study, sage extract significantly inhibited HIV activity by preventing the virus from entering target cells.

Sage has also been shown to combat HSV-1 and Indiana vesiculovirus, which infects farm animals like horses, cows, and pigs.

23. Basil

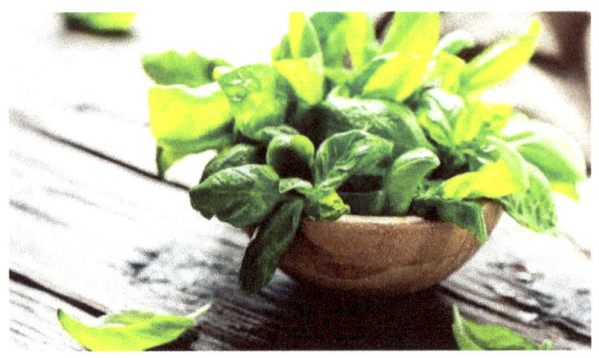

Many types of basil, including the sweet and holy varieties, may fight certain viral infections. For example, one test-tube study found that sweet basil extracts, including compounds like apigenin and ursolic acid, exhibited potent effects against herpes viruses, hepatitis B, and enterovirus.

Holy basil, also known as tulsi, has been shown to increase immunity, which may help fight viral infections.

In a 4-week study in 24 healthy adults, supplementing with 300 mg of holy basil extract significantly increased levels of helper T cells and natural killer cells, both of which are immune cells that help protect and defend your body from viral infections.

24. Fennel

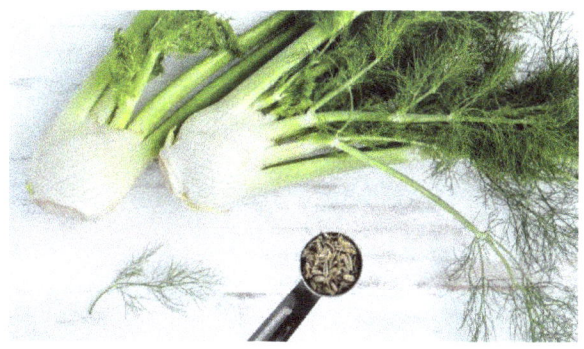

Fennel is a licorice-flavored plant that may fight certain viruses. A test-tube study showed that fennel extract exhibited strong antiviral effects against herpes viruses and parainfluenza type-3 (PI-3), which causes respiratory infections in cattle.

What's more, trans-anethole, the main component of fennel essential oil, has demonstrated powerful antiviral effects against herpes viruses.

According to animal research, fennel may also boost your immune system and decrease inflammation, which may likewise help combat viral infections.

25. Watermelon

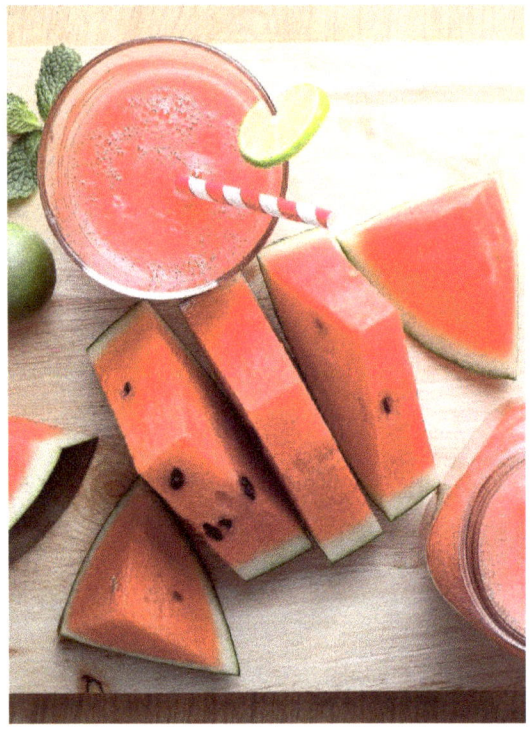

Watermelon juices are best if you have flu or a cold, but it also does the perfect job for boosting your immune system.

Since watermelon helps relieve muscle soreness which is a common symptom found in older adults.

Moreover, it contains Vitamins A and C along with magnesium and zinc which are extremely useful for the body.

26. Tomatoes

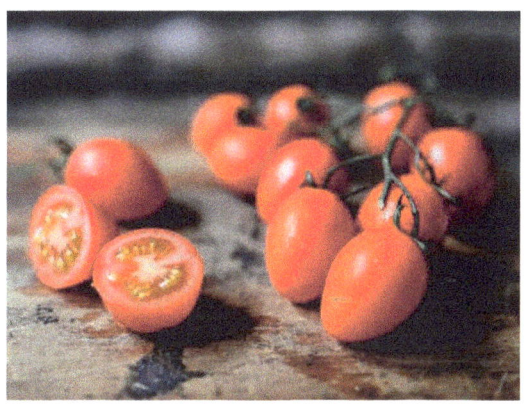

Tomatoes are a great food to eat when you're sick due to their high concentration of vitamin C. Just one medium tomato contains more than 16 milligrams of vitamin C, which is a proven fuel to your body's immune system.

In a German study published by *Medizinische Monatsschrift fur Pharmazeuten*, vitamin C was shown to be a vital part of the strength of the body's phagocytes and t-cells, two major components of the immune system.

The researchers also noted that a deficiency in this nutrient can lead to a weaker immune system and lower resistance to certain pathogens that can lead to illness.

27. Rosemary

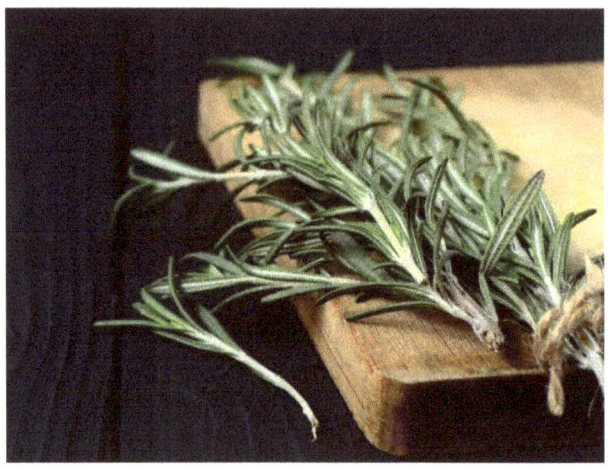

Rosemary isn't just a tasty herb to add to baked goods — it's also an amazing anti-inflammatory and is a rich source of antioxidants. Critical Reviews in Food Science and Nutrition noted that most herbs, such as rosemary.

Contain antioxidants that serve as anti-inflammatory properties in the body. This anti-inflammatory effect allows for better digestive and gut health, leading to a boost in your immune system to keep you healthy.

28. Raw Honey

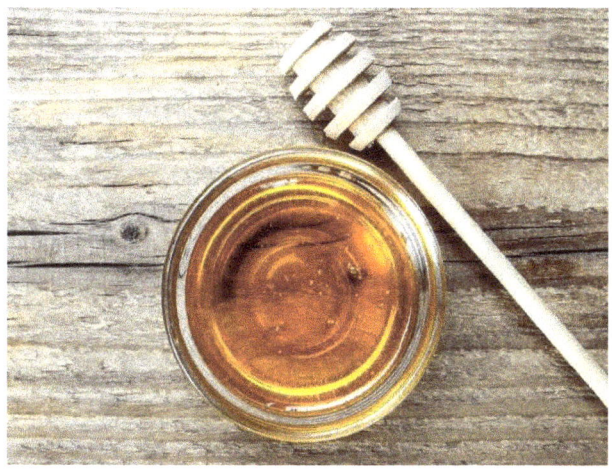

All-natural, raw honey not only tastes delicious but can also help soothe some symptoms of a cold.

Honey is helpful in relieving sore and itchy throats, according to a study published in the *Iran Journal of Basic Medical Science*.

The study also states that honey acts as an antibacterial, killing any germs in the body that can cause you to get sick.

29. Nuts

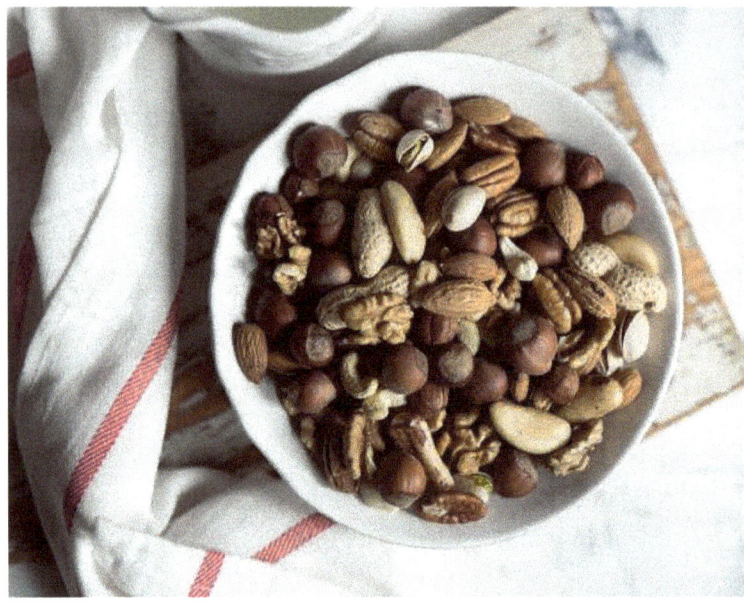

Most nuts contain vitamin E, another vitamin that's crucial to fighting off sickness. A study published in the *Journal of the American College of Nutrition* found that taking 50 milligrams of vitamin E daily helped cigarette-smoking men.

Who were 65 years and older living in cities reduce their risk of catching a cold by 28 percent. However, the researchers noted that more studies need to be conducted in order to fully validate vitamin E's potential in preventing colds.

30. Manggo

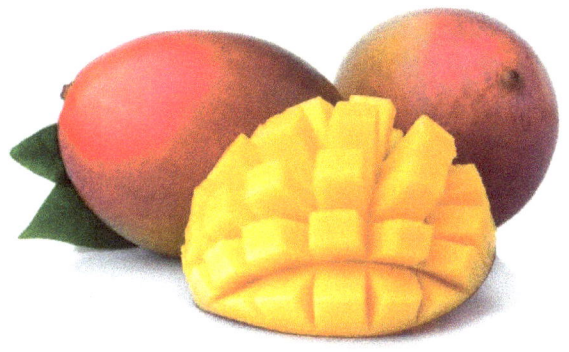

In some parts of the world, mango (*Mangifera indica*) is called the "king of fruits." It's a drupe, or stone fruit, which means that it has a large seed in the middle.

Mango is native to India and Southeast Asia and has been cultivated for over 4,000 years. There are hundreds of types of mango, each with a unique taste, shape, size and color

This fruit is not only delicious but also boasts an impressive nutritional profile.

In fact, studies link mango and its nutrients to health benefits, such as improved immunity, digestive health and eyesight, as well as a lower risk of certain cancers.

Medicinal Herbs to Boosts Immune System Germany Version

Wenn Sie Ihren Körper mit bestimmten Lebensmitteln wie Obst und Gemüse füttern, kann dies dazu beitragen, Ihr Immunsystem zu stärken. Wenn Sie nach Möglichkeiten suchen, um Erkältungen im Winter, Virenbefall und Grippe vorzubeugen.

Ihr erster Schritt sollte ein Besuch in Ihrem örtlichen Lebensmittelgeschäft sein. Planen Sie Ihre Mahlzeiten mit diesen leistungsstarken Boostern des Immunsystems.

1. Zitrusfrüchte

Die meisten Menschen wenden sich nach einer Erkältung Vitamin C zu. Das liegt daran, dass es hilft, Ihr Immunsystem aufzubauen. Es wird angenommen, dass Vitamin C die Produktion weißer Blutkörperchen erhöht. Dies ist der Schlüssel zur Bekämpfung von Infektionen.

Da Ihr Körper es nicht produziert oder speichert, benötigen Sie täglich Vitamin C für eine anhaltende Gesundheit. Fast alle Zitrusfrüchte enthalten viel Vitamin C. Mit einer solchen Auswahl ist es einfach, jeder Mahlzeit einen Spritzer dieses Vitamins hinzuzufügen.

2. Rote Paprika

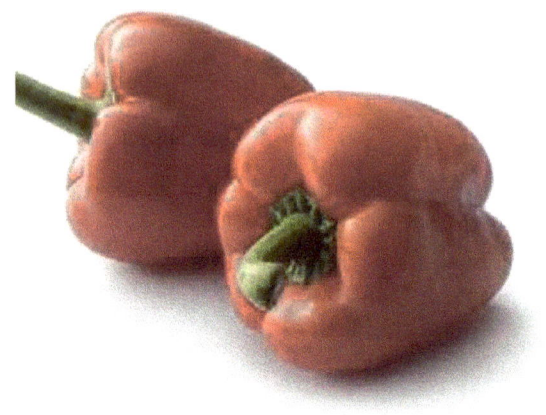

Wenn Sie der Meinung sind, dass Zitrusfrüchte das meiste Vitamin C von Obst oder Gemüse enthalten, denken Sie noch einmal darüber nach. Unze für Unze enthalten rote Paprika doppelt so viel Vitamin C wie Zitrusfrüchte. Sie sind auch eine reichhaltige Quelle für Beta-Carotin.

Vitamin C stärkt nicht nur das Immunsystem, sondern trägt auch zur Erhaltung einer gesunden Haut bei. Beta-Carotin hilft, Ihre Augen und Haut gesund zu halten.

3. Brokkoli

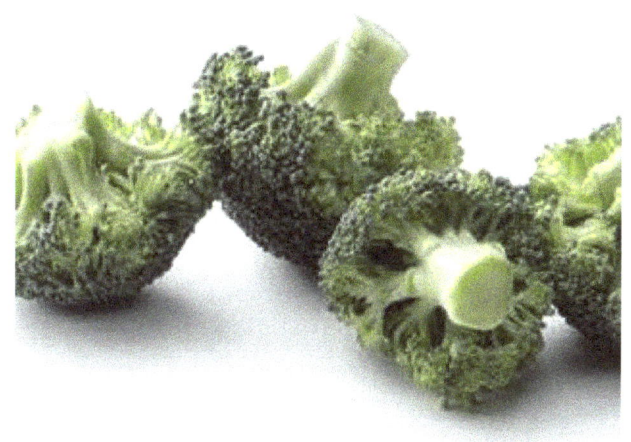

Brokkoli ist mit Vitaminen und Mineralstoffen aufgeladen. Mit den Vitaminen A, C und E sowie vielen anderen Antioxidantien und Ballaststoffen ist Brokkoli eines der gesündesten Gemüse, die Sie auf Ihren Tisch legen können.

Der Schlüssel, um seine Kraft intakt zu halten, besteht darin, es so wenig wie möglich zu kochen - oder noch besser, überhaupt nicht.

4. Knoblauch

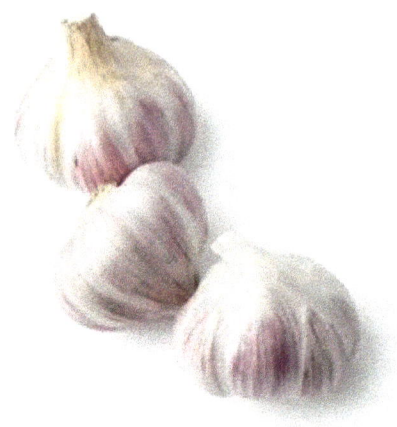

Knoblauch ist in fast jeder Küche der Welt zu finden. Es verleiht dem Essen ein wenig Schwung und ist ein Muss für Ihre Gesundheit. Frühe Zivilisationen erkannten ihren Wert bei der Bekämpfung von Infektionen.

Laut dem Nationalen Zentrum für Komplementär und Integrativ kann Knoblauch auch dazu beitragen, den Blutdruck zu senken und die Verhärtung der Arterien zu verlangsamen.

Die immunstärkenden Eigenschaften von Knoblauch scheinen von einer hohen Konzentration schwefelhaltiger Verbindungen wie Allicin zu stammen.

5. Ingwer

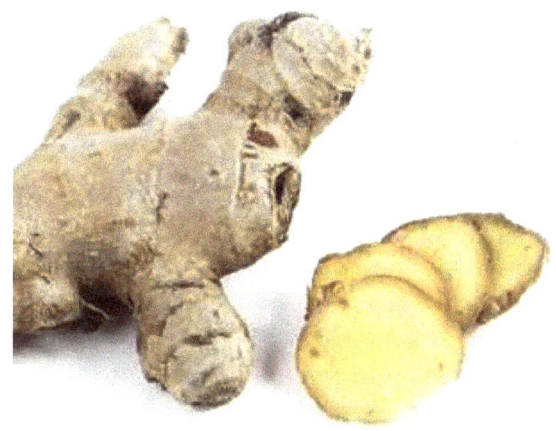

Ingwer ist eine weitere Zutat, an die sich viele wenden, nachdem sie krank geworden sind. Ingwer kann helfen, Entzündungen zu lindern, was Halsschmerzen und andere entzündliche Erkrankungen lindern kann. Ingwer kann auch helfen, Übelkeit zu verringern.

Während es in vielen süßen Desserts verwendet wird, packt Ingwer etwas Wärme in Form von Gingerol, einem Verwandten von Capsaicin. Ingwer kann helfen, chronische Schmerzen zu lindern, und kann laut jüngsten Tierversuchen cholesterinsenkende Eigenschaften besitzen.

6. Spinat

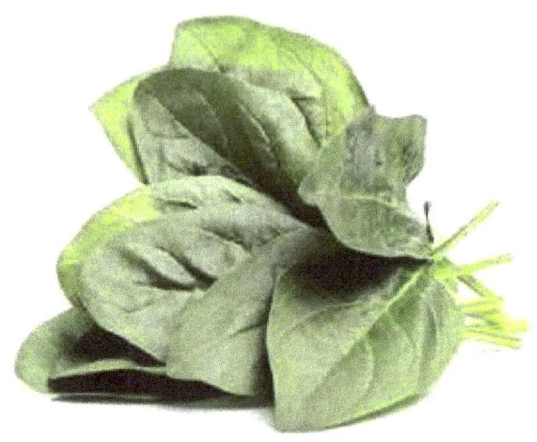

Spinat wurde nicht nur deshalb auf unsere Liste gesetzt, weil er reich an Vitamin C ist. Er enthält auch zahlreiche Antioxidantien und Beta-Carotin, die die Fähigkeit unseres Immunsystems zur Infektionsbekämpfung verbessern können.

Ähnlich wie Brokkoli ist Spinat am gesündesten, wenn er so wenig wie möglich gekocht wird, damit er seine Nährstoffe behält. Leichtes Kochen erhöht jedoch das Vitamin A und ermöglicht die Freisetzung anderer Nährstoffe aus Oxalsäure.

7. Joghurt

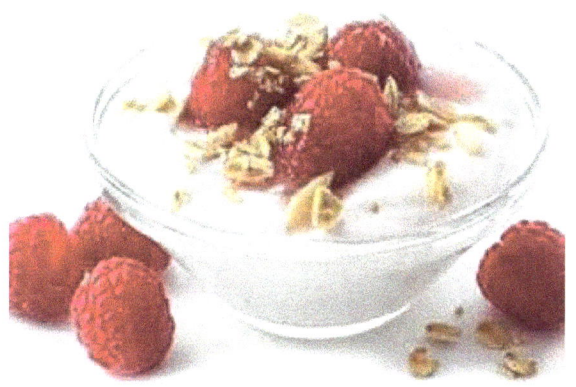

Suchen Sie nach Joghurt, auf dessen Etikett „lebende und aktive Kulturen "aufgedruckt sind, wie z. B. griechischer Joghurt. Diese Kulturen können Ihr Immunsystem stimulieren, um Krankheiten zu bekämpfen.

Versuchen Sie, einfachen Joghurt zu bekommen, anstatt die Sorten, die vorgeschmackt und mit Zucker beladen sind.

Sie können Naturjoghurt stattdessen selbst mit gesunden Früchten und einem Spritzer Honig süßen.

Joghurt kann auch eine großartige Quelle für Vitamin D sein. Versuchen Sie daher, mit Vitamin D angereicherte Marken auszuwählen.

Vitamin D hilft bei der Regulierung des Immunsystems und soll die natürlichen Abwehrkräfte unseres Körpers gegen Krankheiten stärken.

8. Mandeln

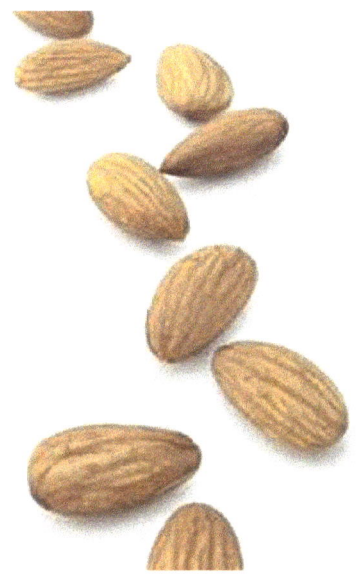

Wenn es darum geht, Erkältungen vorzubeugen und sie abzuwehren, tritt Vitamin E tendenziell in den Hintergrund von Vitamin C.

Vitamin E ist jedoch der Schlüssel zu einem gesunden Immunsystem. Es ist ein fettlösliches Vitamin, was bedeutet, dass Fett vorhanden sein muss, um richtig aufgenommen zu werden.

Nüsse wie Mandeln sind mit dem Vitamin gefüllt und haben auch gesunde Fette. Eine halbe Tasse Portion, die etwa 46 ganze, geschälte Mandeln enthält, liefert fast 100 Prozent der empfohlenen täglichen Menge an Vitamin E.

9. Kurkuma

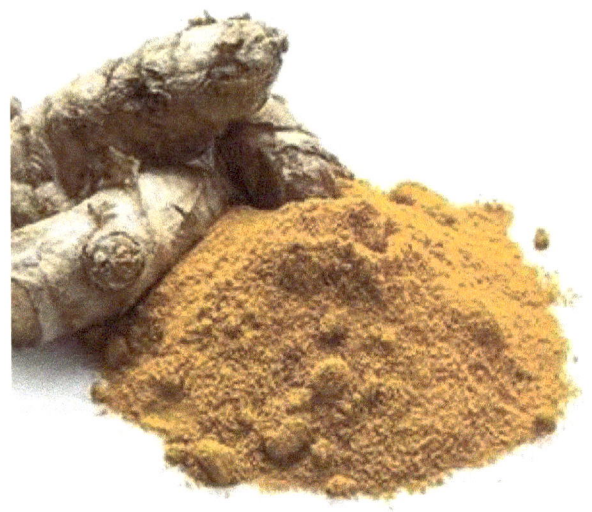

Sie kennen Kurkuma als Hauptbestandteil in vielen Currys. Dieses leuchtend gelbe, bittere Gewürz wird aber auch seit Jahren als entzündungshemmendes Mittel bei der Behandlung von Arthrose und rheumatoider Arthritis eingesetzt.

Untersuchungen zeigen auch, dass hohe Curcumin-Konzentrationen, die Kurkuma seine charakteristische Farbe verleihen, dazu beitragen können, durch körperliche Betätigung verursachte Muskelschäden zu verringern.

10. Grüner Tee

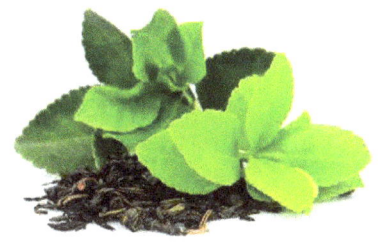

Sowohl grüne als auch schwarze Tees sind mit Flavonoiden gefüllt, einer Art Antioxidans. Wo grüner Tee wirklich herausragend ist, ist sein Gehalt an Epigallocatechingallat oder EGCG, einem weiteren starken Antioxidans. Es wurde gezeigt, dass EGCG die Immunfunktion verbessert.

Der Fermentationsprozess von schwarzem Tee zerstört einen Großteil des EGCG. Grüner Tee hingegen wird gedämpft und nicht fermentiert, so dass das EGCG erhalten bleibt.

Grüner Tee ist auch eine gute Quelle für die Aminosäure L-Theanin. L-Theanin kann die Produktion von keimbekämpfenden Verbindungen in Ihren T-Zellen unterstützen.

11. Papaya

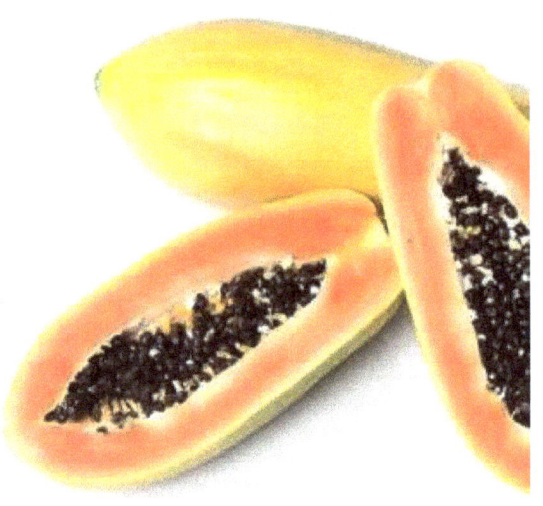

Papaya ist eine weitere Frucht, die mit Vitamin C beladen ist. In einer einzigen Papaya finden Sie 224 Prozent der täglich empfohlenen Menge an Vitamin C.

Papayas haben auch ein Verdauungsenzym namens Papain, das entzündungshemmende Wirkungen hat.

Papayas haben anständige Mengen an Kalium, B-Vitaminen und Folsäure, die alle für Ihre allgemeine Gesundheit von Vorteil sind.

12. Kiwi

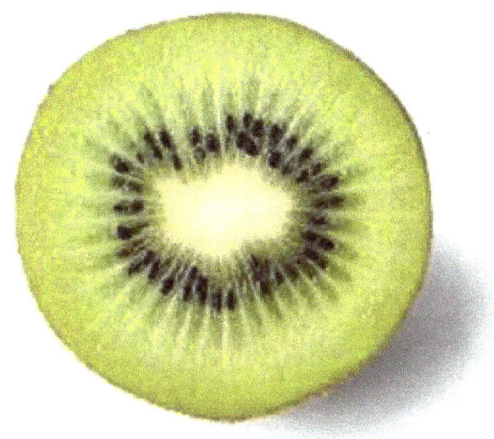

Wie Papayas enthalten Kiwis von Natur aus eine Menge essentieller Nährstoffe, darunter Folsäure, Kalium, Vitamin K und Vitamin C.

Vitamin C stärkt die weißen Blutkörperchen, um Infektionen zu bekämpfen, während die anderen Nährstoffe von Kiwi dafür sorgen, dass der Rest Ihres Körpers ordnungsgemäß funktioniert.

13. Sonnenblumenkerne

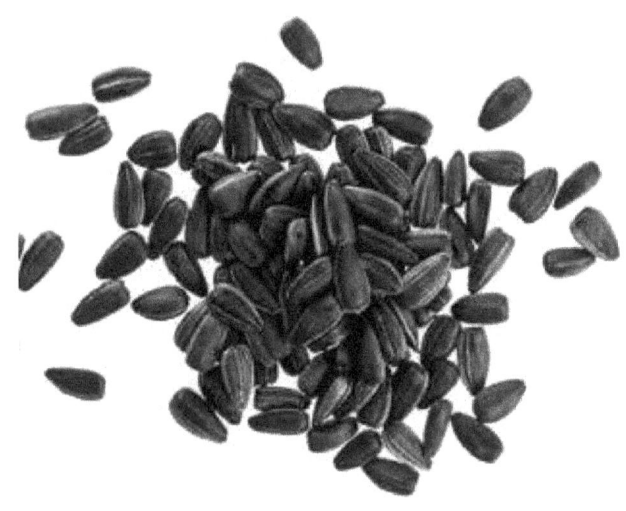

Sonnenblumenkerne sind voller Nährstoffe, darunter Phosphor, Magnesium und Vitamin B-6. Sie sind auch unglaublich reich an Vitamin E, einem starken Antioxidans.

Vitamin E ist wichtig für die Regulierung und Aufrechterhaltung der Funktion des Immunsystems. Andere Lebensmittel mit hohen Mengen an Vitamin E sind Avocados und dunkles Blattgemüse.

14. Oregano

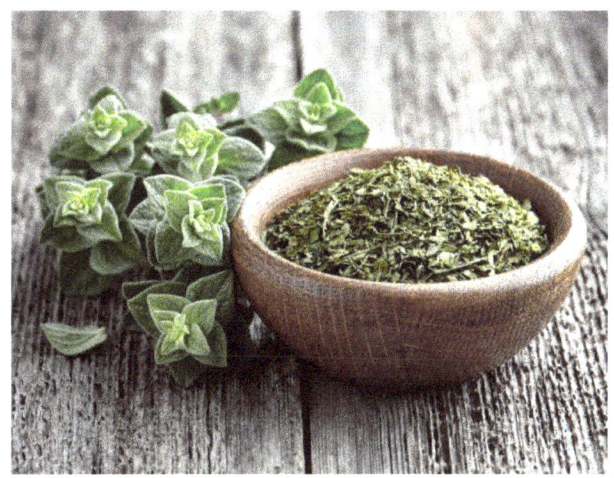

Oregano ist ein beliebtes Kraut in der Familie der Minzen, das für seine beeindruckenden medizinischen Eigenschaften bekannt ist. Seine Pflanzenstoffe, zu denen Carvacrol gehört, bieten antivirale Eigenschaften.

In einer Reagenzglasstudie reduzierten sowohl Oreganoöl als auch isoliertes Carvacrol die Aktivität des murinen Norovirus (MNV) innerhalb von 15 Minuten nach Exposition.

MNV ist hoch ansteckend und die Hauptursache für die Magengrippe beim Menschen. Es ist dem humanen Norovirus sehr ähnlich und wird in wissenschaftlichen Studien verwendet, da es bekanntermaßen schwierig ist, das humane Norovirus in Laborumgebungen zu züchten

Es wurde auch gezeigt, dass Oreganoöl und Carvacrol eine antivirale Aktivität gegen Herpes-simplex-Virus Typ-1 (HSV-1) zeigen; Rotavirus, eine häufige Ursache für Durchfall bei Säuglingen und Kindern; und Respiratory Syncytial Virus (RSV), das Infektionen der Atemwege verursacht.

15. Echinacea

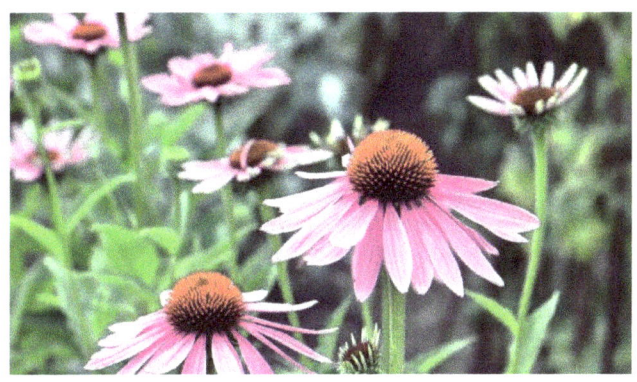

Echinacea ist aufgrund seiner beeindruckenden gesundheitsfördernden Eigenschaften einer der am häufigsten verwendeten Inhaltsstoffe in der Kräutermedizin. Viele Teile der Pflanze, einschließlich ihrer Blüten, Blätter und Wurzeln, werden für natürliche Heilmittel verwendet.

Tatsächlich wurde Echinacea purpurea, eine Sorte, die kegelförmige Blüten hervorbringt, von amerikanischen Ureinwohnern zur Behandlung einer Vielzahl von Erkrankungen, einschließlich Virusinfektionen, verwendet.

Mehrere Reagenzglasstudien legen nahe, dass bestimmte Sorten von Echinacea, einschließlich E. pallida, E. angustifolia und E. purpurea, besonders wirksam bei der Bekämpfung von Virusinfektionen wie Herpes und Influenza sind.

Insbesondere wird angenommen, dass E. purpurea auch eine immunverstärkende Wirkung hat, was es besonders nützlich für die Behandlung von Virusinfektionen macht.

16. Ginseng

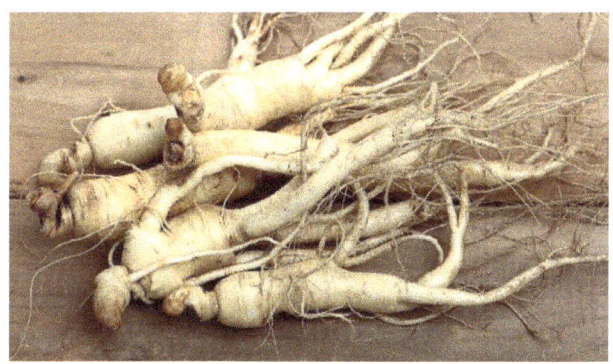

Ginseng, das in koreanischen und amerikanischen Sorten vorkommt, ist die Wurzel der Pflanzen der Familie Panax. Es wurde lange Zeit in der traditionellen chinesischen Medizin eingesetzt und hat sich als besonders wirksam bei der Bekämpfung von Viren erwiesen.

In Tier- und Reagenzglasstudien hat der koreanische rote Ginseng-Extrakt signifikante Wirkungen gegen RSV, Herpesviren und Hepatitis A gezeigt.

Außerdem haben Verbindungen in Ginseng, die als Ginsenoside bezeichnet werden, antivirale Wirkungen gegen Hepatitis B, Norovirus und Coxsackieviren, die mit mehreren schwerwiegenden Krankheiten verbunden sind - einschließlich einer Infektion des Gehirns, die als Meningoenzephalitis bezeichnet wird.

17. Pfefferminze

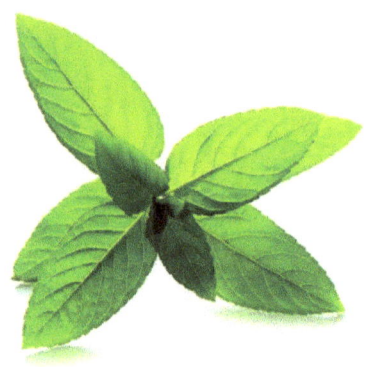

Pfefferminze hat bekanntermaßen starke antivirale Eigenschaften und wird üblicherweise Tees, Extrakten und Tinkturen zugesetzt, die zur natürlichen Behandlung von Virusinfektionen bestimmt sind.

Seine Blätter und ätherischen Öle enthalten Wirkstoffe wie Menthol und Rosmarinsäure, die antiviral und entzündungshemmend wirken.

18. Sambucus

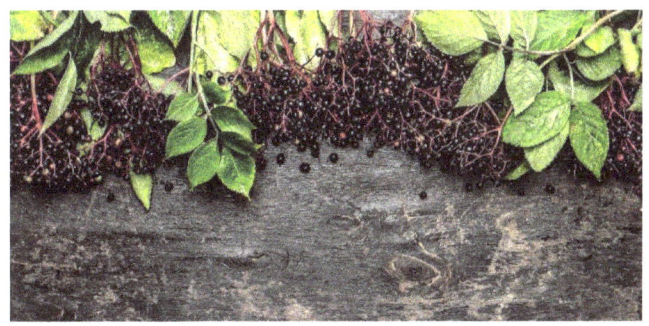

Sambucus ist eine Pflanzenfamilie, die auch Holunder genannt wird. Holunderbeeren werden zu einer Vielzahl von Produkten verarbeitet, wie Elixieren und Pillen, die zur natürlichen Behandlung von Virusinfektionen wie Grippe und Erkältung verwendet werden.

Eine Studie an Mäusen ergab, dass konzentrierter Holundersaft die Replikation des Influenzavirus unterdrückte und die Reaktion des Immunsystems stimulierte.

Darüber hinaus wurde in einer Überprüfung von 4 Studien an 180 Personen festgestellt, dass Holunderpräparate die durch Virusinfektionen verursachten Symptome der oberen Atemwege erheblich reduzieren.

19. Süßholz

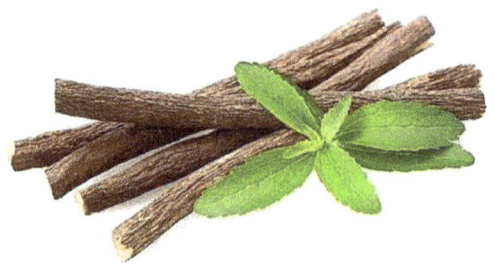

Süßholz wird seit Jahrhunderten in der traditionellen chinesischen Medizin und anderen natürlichen Praktiken verwendet. Glycyrrhizin, Liquiritigenin und Glabridin sind nur einige der Wirkstoffe in Süßholz, die starke antivirale Eigenschaften haben.

Reagenzglasstudien zeigen, dass Süßholzwurzelextrakt gegen HIV, RSV, Herpesviren und schweres Coronavirus (SARS-CoV) im Zusammenhang mit dem akuten respiratorischen Syndrom wirksam ist, das eine schwere Art von Lungenentzündung verursacht.

20. Astragalus

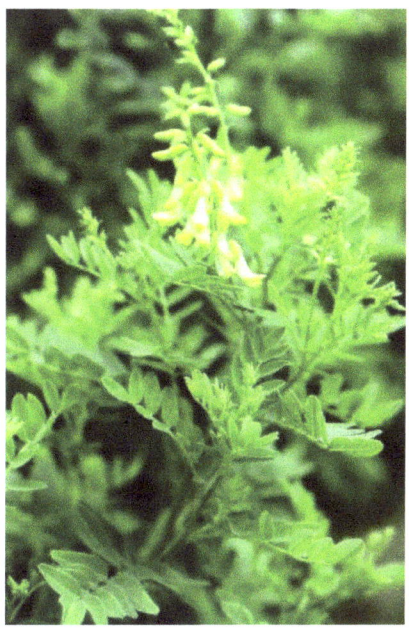

Astragalus ist ein blühendes Kraut, das in der traditionellen chinesischen Medizin beliebt ist. Es verfügt über Astragalus-Polysaccharid (APS), das signifikante immunverstärkende und antivirale Eigenschaften aufweist.

Reagenzglas- und Tierstudien zeigen, dass Astragalus Herpesviren, Hepatitis C und das Vogelgrippe-H9-Virus bekämpft.Außerdem legen Reagenzglasstudien nahe, dass APS menschliche Astrozytenzellen, den am häufigsten vorkommenden Zelltyp im Zentralnervensystem, vor einer Infektion mit Herpes schützen kann.

21. Löwenzahn

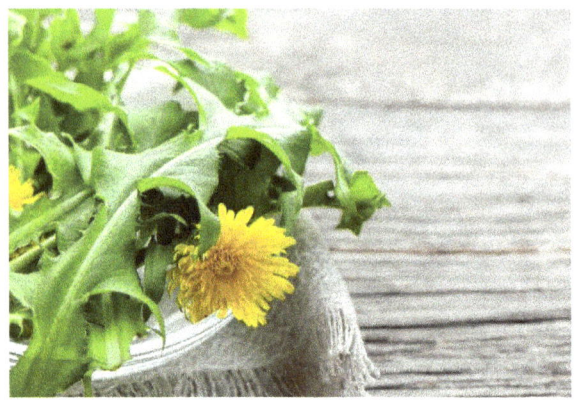

Löwenzahn wird allgemein als Unkraut angesehen, wurde jedoch auf verschiedene medizinische Eigenschaften untersucht, einschließlich möglicher antiviraler Wirkungen. Reagenzglasuntersuchungen zeigen, dass Löwenzahn Hepatitis B, HIV und Influenza bekämpfen kann.

Darüber hinaus wurde in einer Reagenzglasstudie festgestellt, dass Löwenzahnextrakt die Replikation von Dengue-Fieber hemmt, einem von Mücken übertragenen Virus, das Dengue-Fieber verursacht.

Diese Krankheit, die tödlich sein kann, löst Symptome wie hohes Fieber, Erbrechen und Muskelschmerzen aus.

22. Salbei

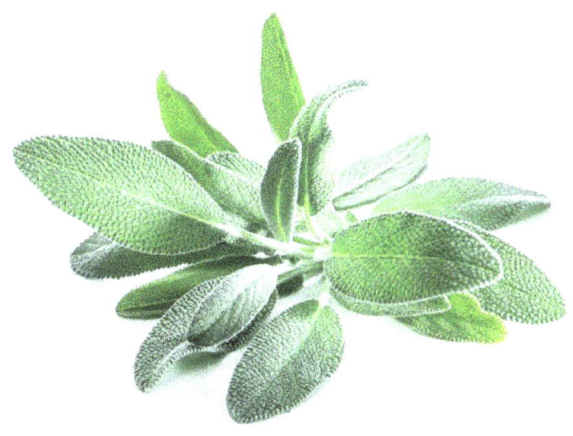

Salbei gehört ebenfalls zur Familie der Minzen und ist ein aromatisches Kraut, das in der traditionellen Medizin seit langem zur Behandlung von Virusinfektionen verwendet wird.

Die antiviralen Eigenschaften von Salbei werden hauptsächlich auf Verbindungen namens Safficinolid und Salbei zurückgeführt, die in den Blättern und im Stamm der Pflanze vorkommen.

Reagenzglasuntersuchungen zeigen, dass dieses Kraut das humane Immundefizienzvirus Typ 1 (HIV-1) bekämpfen kann, das zu AIDS führen kann. In einer Studie hemmte Salbei-Extrakt die HIV-Aktivität signifikant, indem er das Eindringen des Virus in Zielzellen verhinderte. Es wurde auch gezeigt, dass Salbei HSV-1 und Indiana Vesiculovirus bekämpft, das Nutztiere wie Pferde, Kühe und Schweine infiziert.

23. Basil

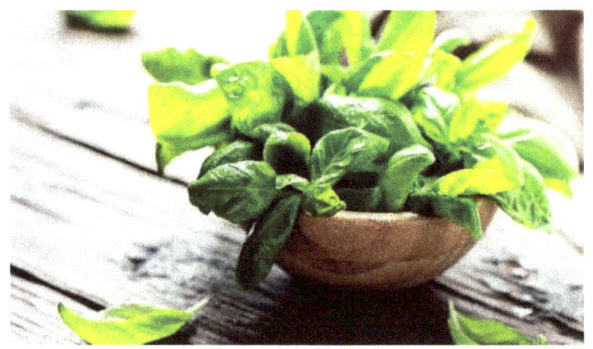

Viele Arten von Basilikum, einschließlich der süßen und heiligen Sorten, können bestimmte Virusinfektionen bekämpfen. Beispielsweise ergab eine Reagenzglasstudie, dass Extrakte aus süßem Basilikum, einschließlich Verbindungen wie Apigenin und Ursolsäure, starke Wirkungen gegen Herpesviren, Hepatitis B und Enterovirus zeigten.

Es wurde gezeigt, dass heiliges Basilikum, auch als Tulsi bekannt, die Immunität erhöht, was zur Bekämpfung von Virusinfektionen beitragen kann.

In einer 4-wöchigen Studie an 24 gesunden Erwachsenen erhöhte die Ergänzung mit 300 mg Heilig-Basilikum-Extrakt die Spiegel an Helfer-T-Zellen und natürlichen Killerzellen, die beide Immunzellen sind, die Ihren Körper vor Virusinfektionen schützen und verteidigen.

24. Fenchel

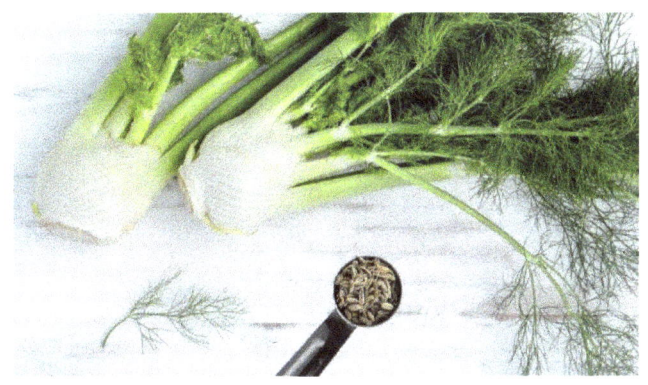

Fenchel ist eine Pflanze mit Lakritzgeschmack, die bestimmte Viren bekämpfen kann. Eine Reagenzglasstudie zeigte, dass Fenchelextrakt starke antivirale Wirkungen gegen Herpesviren und Parainfluenza Typ-3 (PI-3) zeigte, die bei Rindern Infektionen der Atemwege verursachen.

Darüber hinaus hat Transanethol, der Hauptbestandteil des ätherischen Fenchelöls, starke antivirale Wirkungen gegen Herpesviren gezeigt.

Laut Tierversuchen kann Fenchel auch Ihr Immunsystem stärken und Entzündungen verringern, was ebenfalls zur Bekämpfung von Virusinfektionen beitragen kann.

25. Wassermelone

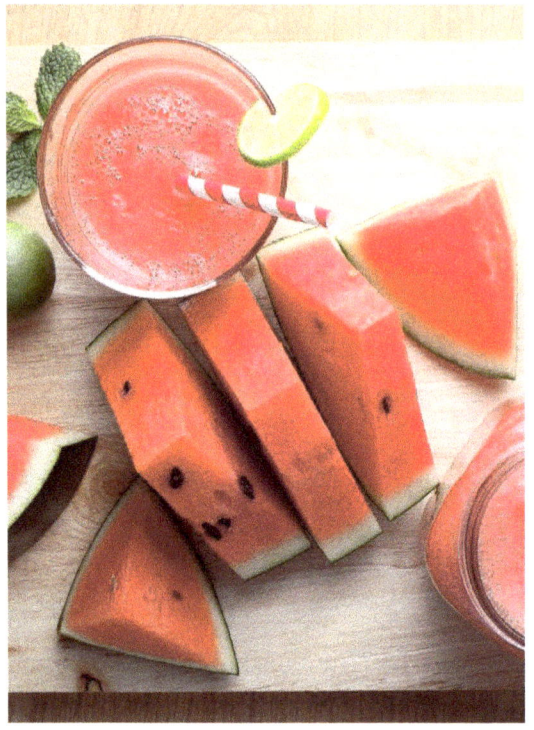

Wassermelonensäfte sind am besten geeignet, wenn Sie an Grippe oder Erkältung leiden, aber sie eignen sich auch perfekt zur Stärkung Ihres Immunsystems.

Da Wassermelone hilft, Muskelkater zu lindern, ist ein häufiges Symptom bei älteren Erwachsenen.

Darüber hinaus enthält es die Vitamine A und C sowie Magnesium und Zink, die für den Körper äußerst nützlich sind.

26. Tomaten

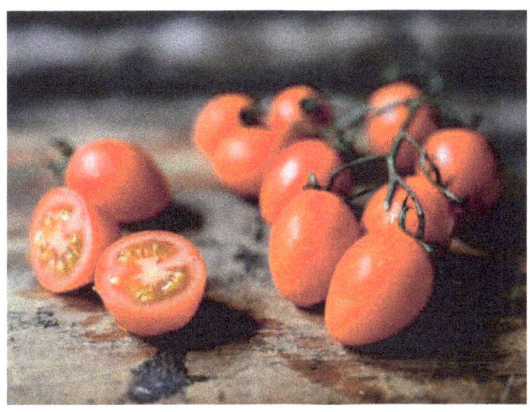

Tomaten sind aufgrund ihrer hohen Vitamin C-Konzentration ein großartiges Lebensmittel, wenn Sie krank sind. Nur eine mittlere Tomate enthält mehr als 16 Milligramm Vitamin C, ein bewährter Kraftstoff für das Immunsystem Ihres Körpers.

In einer deutschen Studie der Medizinischen Monatsschrift für Pharmazeuten wurde gezeigt, dass Vitamin C ein wesentlicher Bestandteil der Stärke der Phagozyten und T-Zellen des Körpers ist, zwei Hauptkomponenten des Immunsystems.

Die Forscher stellten außerdem fest, dass ein Mangel an diesem Nährstoff zu einem schwächeren Immunsystem und einer geringeren Resistenz gegen bestimmte Krankheitserreger führen kann, die zu Krankheiten führen können.

27. Rosmarin

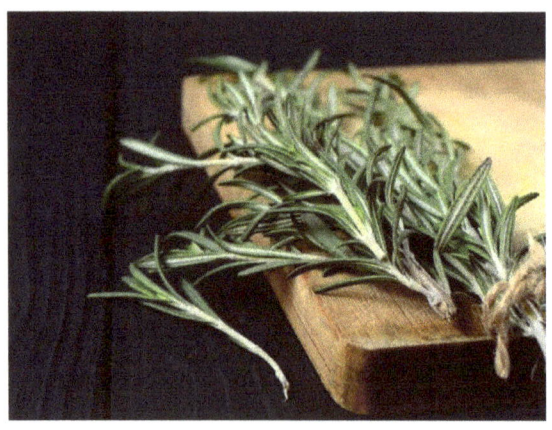

Rosmarin ist nicht nur ein leckeres Kraut für Backwaren, sondern auch ein erstaunliches entzündungshemmendes Mittel und eine reichhaltige Quelle an Antioxidantien. Kritische Bewertungen in Lebensmittelwissenschaft und Ernährung stellten fest, dass die meisten Kräuter, wie Rosmarin.

Enthalten Antioxidantien, die als entzündungshemmende Eigenschaften im Körper dienen. Diese entzündungshemmende Wirkung sorgt für eine bessere Verdauungs- und Darmgesundheit und führt zu einer Stärkung Ihres Immunsystems, um gesund zu bleiben.

28. Roher Honig

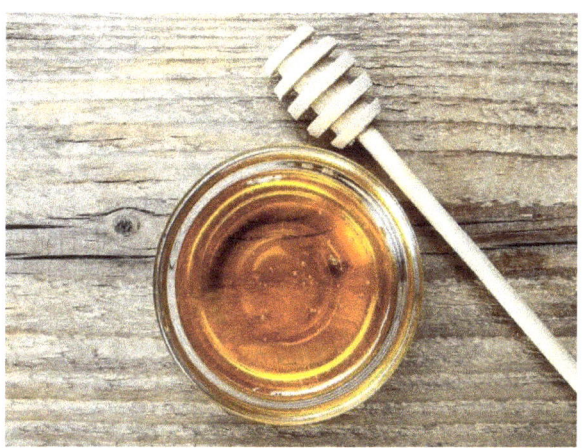

Natürlicher, roher Honig schmeckt nicht nur köstlich, sondern kann auch dazu beitragen, einige Erkältungssymptome zu lindern.

Laut einer im Iran Journal of Basic Medical Science veröffentlichten Studie ist Honig hilfreich bei der Linderung von Halsschmerzen und Juckreiz.

Die Studie besagt auch, dass Honig als antibakterielles Mittel wirkt und alle Keime im Körper abtötet, die dazu führen können, dass Sie krank werden.

29. Muttern

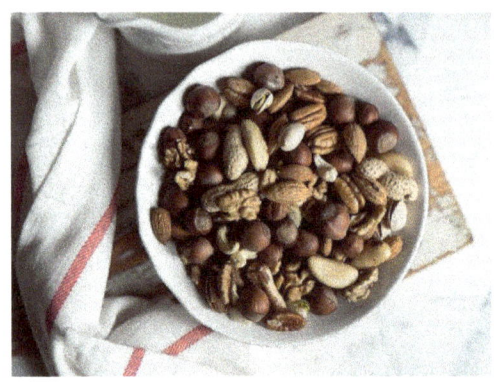

Die meisten Nüsse enthalten Vitamin E, ein weiteres Vitamin, das für die Bekämpfung von Krankheiten von entscheidender Bedeutung ist.

Eine im Journal des American College of Nutrition veröffentlichte Studie ergab, dass die tägliche Einnahme von 50 Milligramm Vitamin E Männern hilft, die Zigaretten rauchen.

Personen ab 65 Jahren, die in Städten leben, reduzieren ihr Erkältungsrisiko um 28 Prozent. Die Forscher stellten jedoch fest, dass weitere Studien durchgeführt werden müssen, um das Potenzial von Vitamin E zur Vorbeugung von Erkältungen vollständig zu validieren.

30. Manggo

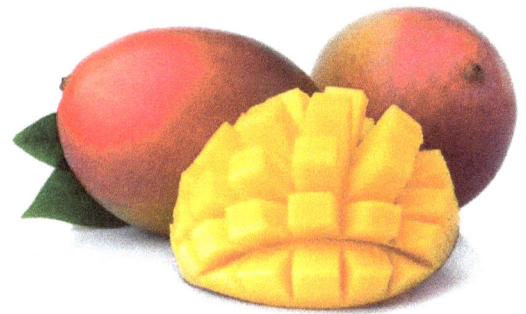

In einigen Teilen der Welt wird Mango (Mangifera indica) als „König der Früchte" bezeichnet. Es ist eine Steinfrucht oder Steinobst, was bedeutet, dass es einen großen Samen in der Mitte hat.

Mango stammt aus Indien und Südostasien und wird seit über 4.000 Jahren angebaut. Es gibt Hunderte von Mangosorten, jede mit einem einzigartigen Geschmack, Form, Größe und Farbe

Diese Frucht ist nicht nur köstlich, sondern weist auch ein beeindruckendes Ernährungsprofil auf.

Tatsächlich verbinden Studien Mango und ihre Nährstoffe mit gesundheitlichen Vorteilen wie einer verbesserten Immunität, Verdauungsgesundheit und Sehkraft sowie einem geringeren Risiko für bestimmte Krebsarten.

Lightning Source UK Ltd.
Milton Keynes UK
UKHW021830080121
376661UK00001B/43